Urinary Tract Infection Diet

A Beginner's 4-Step Guide for Women on Managing UTI Through Diet, With Sample Curated Recipes

mf

copyright © 2022 Mary Golanna

All rights reserved No part of this book may be reproduced, or stored in a retrieval system, or transmitted in any form or by any means, electronic, mechanical, photocopying, recording, or otherwise, without express written permission of the publisher.

Disclaimer

By reading this disclaimer, you are accepting the terms of the disclaimer in full. If you disagree with this disclaimer, please do not read the guide.

All of the content within this guide is provided for informational and educational purposes only, and should not be accepted as independent medical or other professional advice. The author is not a doctor, physician, nurse, mental health provider, or registered nutritionist/dietician. Therefore, using and reading this guide does not establish any form of a physician-patient relationship.

Always consult with a physician or another qualified health provider with any issues or questions you might have regarding any sort of medical condition. Do not ever disregard any qualified professional medical advice or delay seeking that advice because of anything you have read in this guide. The information in this guide is not intended to be any sort of medical advice and should not be used in lieu of any medical advice by a licensed and qualified medical professional.

The information in this guide has been compiled from a variety of known sources. However, the author cannot attest to or guarantee the accuracy of each source and thus should not be held liable for any errors or omissions.

You acknowledge that the publisher of this guide will not be held liable for any loss or damage of any kind incurred as a result of this guide or the reliance on any information provided within this guide. You acknowledge and agree that you assume all risk and responsibility for any action you undertake in response to the information in this guide.

Using this guide does not guarantee any particular result (e.g., weight loss or a cure). By reading this guide, you acknowledge that there are no guarantees to any specific outcome or results you can expect.

All product names, diet plans, or names used in this guide are for identification purposes only and are the property of their respective owners. The use of these names does not imply endorsement. All other trademarks cited herein are the property of their respective owners.

Where applicable, this guide is not intended to be a substitute for the original work of this diet plan and is, at most, a supplement to the original work for this diet plan and never a direct substitute. This guide is a personal expression of the facts of that diet plan.

Where applicable, persons shown in the cover images are stock photography models and the publisher has obtained the rights to use the images through license agreements with third-party stock image companies.

Table of Contents

Introduction   7
All About Urinary Tract Infection (UTI)   9
    What are some common symptoms?   9
    What causes urinary tract infections?   10
    What are some reasons for this?   11
    Are there certain risk factors for UTIs?   12
Diagnosing, Management, and Prevention of UTIs   13
    Diagnosis   13
    How do you treat UTIs?   14
    What about alternative treatments for UTIs?   15
    Is there a way to prevent UTIs?   16
The UTI Diet   18
    The most common UTI-triggering foods are (and thus should be avoided):   19
    These are some good foods to eat: 20
Your 4-Step Plan for Managing UTIs   24
    Step 1: Keep your bladder healthy   24
    Step 2: Prevent bacteria from building up in your urinary tract   25
    Step 3: Manage urinary tract infections   26
    Step 4: Eat a UTI-friendly Diet   27
Sample Recipes   28
    Garlic Broccoli Salad   29
    Grenade Salad   30
    Spinach and Watercress Salad   31
    Kale Salad with Strawberry and Almonds   32
    Roasted Veggies   33
    Coleslaw   34
    Seafood Stew   35

Baked Tuna and Asparagus	36
Baked Salmon	37
Garbanzo-Kale and Butternut Squash Burger	38
Lentil Soup	39
Vegetable Broth	41
Zucchini and Celery Greens Soup	43
Energy Oats	45
Spinach Quiche	46
Salmon and Fennel Salad	48
Marinated Tuna Steak	50
Creamy Low-FODMAP Fish Casserole	51
Conclusion	**53**
References and Helpful Links	**54**

Introduction

Urinary tract infections, or UTIs, are reported among the most common diseases and facts show that each year 1 in 4 women will suffer from a UTI, and 30 to 50 percent of these patients will have a recurrence.

UTIs are caused by bacteria that infect the urinary tract. The infection can be limited to the bladder (cystitis) or affect the kidneys (nephritis) if it travels up the ureters.

We've seen how medical doctors deal with this, but did you know there is another option? Diet can have a great impact on your immune system which makes it possible to fight off bacteria trying to invade your urinary tract. Not only that, diet can help reduce pain caused by bladder inflammation through anti-inflammatory foods.

In this guide, you will discover:

- The basics behind UTIs
- The most common causes for UTIs, how medical doctors treat them, and what to avoid when you have a UTI

- Alternative options for treating UTIs, and what to eat and avoid when you have a UTI
- The best foods to eat and the worst foods to avoid when you have a UTI
- How to prevent future recurrence of UTIs
- Sample Recipes

All About Urinary Tract Infection (UTI)

A urinary tract infection (UTI) is a type of urinary tract infection that affects the lower part of your urinary tract. This includes your bladder and urethra.

Other types of UTIs are characterized by infections higher up in the urinary system, like the kidneys or ureters; these types are called ascending infections (or pyelonephritis).

It may be caused by bacteria moving up the urinary tract from an infection somewhere else in the body, like your vagina or skin, or it could develop after you've had surgery to remove your bladder.

What are some common symptoms?

The most common symptoms include:

- Frequent urge to urinate
- Painful and burning sensation while urinating
- Blood in urine
- Strong smelling urine

- Painful and enlarged abdomen (rare)
- Symptoms may vary depending on the age of the patient as well as an individual's immune system.

In addition, symptoms can also vary between men and women. For example, in men, the most common symptoms are a burning sensation while urinating or an urgent need to urinate. They do not typically experience pain in their abdomen unless it is caused by another condition such as kidney stones. In women, infections tend to be more severe. Symptoms include fever, chills, back pain, and painful intercourse from vaginal infection.

What causes urinary tract infections?

Bacteria called E. coli found in your intestines may sometimes find their way into your urinary tract through the urethra (opening of the bladder). This is because during bowel movements you flush out bacteria that goes down the urethra when urine exits the bladder through the urethra which therefore makes it easier for harmful bacteria to travel up the urethra.

Pregnancy can also make a woman more prone to UTIs. This is because during pregnancy the growing uterus presses on your bladder making you feel like you want to urinate more frequently, resulting in frequent bacteria exposure that eventually causes an infection.

Some of the most common causes include:

- Frequent bowel movements or diarrhea
- Poor hygiene habits (i.e.: wiping from back to front)
- Wiping after urinating
- Douching/Intimate hygiene products (soaps, vaginal sprays, feminine wipes)
- An uncircumcised penis may cause bacteria to build up under the foreskin or around the tip of the penis which makes it easier for harmful bacteria to enter the urethra when urine passes through the opening of the foreskin while passing

What are some reasons for this?

There are several known causes of urinary tract infections, including:

- Bacteria in the bowel which sometimes avoid being absorbed by the body flow into the bladder
- Problems with the kidney, ureter, or bladder prevent the body from flushing out harmful bacteria. For example, an enlarged prostate can put pressure on the urethra and stop urine flow which in turn helps bad bacteria to travel up the urinary tract.
- Women are more likely than men to experience UTIs because their urethra is shorter than that of a man's, making it easier for bacteria to reach their bladder.

- Diabetes, which results in high levels of sugar in the blood, increases the risk of urinary tract infections by providing additional food for bad bacteria like E. coli to thrive on.

Are there certain risk factors for UTIs?

Several risk factors can affect a woman's chance of getting a UTI. These include:

- Using birth control that contains both estrogen and progesterone
- Using an IUD (intrauterine device) for contraception, which releases the hormone progesterone into the body
- Having sex with multiple partners or a partner who has other sexual partners
- Wiping from back to front after going to the bathroom, may push bacteria toward the urethra and bladder
- Being sexually active. Anyone sexually active, even women in long-term relationships, can get a UTI. This is because the urethra (the tube urine travels through) runs from the bladder to just before the opening of the vagina. During sexual intercourse or any other activity involving direct contact between the urethra and something else, bacteria may be pushed up into the bladder causing an infection.

Diagnosing, Management, and Prevention of UTIs

Diagnosis

A urine test is the best way to find out if you have a UTI. A nurse or doctor will ask for a sample of your urine to see if there are any signs of infection, including white blood cells, bacteria, or nitrites. If these are present, it means an infection is present and treatment may be necessary.

Several tests are used to determine if urinary tract infections are caused by bacteria or other organisms. These may include:

- Urine Culture - This involves checking a sample of your urine for the presence of bacteria and determining which types they are. If you're not prescribed antibiotics, this test is repeated after treatment with medication to see if the antibiotic has been effective in treating your infection and preventing another one from occurring
- Narrow-Spectrum Urine Antibiotic Assay (NAUA) - This allows the doctor to prescribe the most suitable antibiotic for your particular type of UTI. It also tells

the doctor if the medication they are prescribing is working against your urinary tract infection
- Urine Osmolality - This helps determine if there are other factors involved in your UTI, which may include diabetes or kidney disease. Urine osmolality is often tested at the same time as a urine culture

How do you treat UTIs?

UTIs usually go away within a few days when treated but can return if treatment isn't continued properly. Treatment for UTIs varies depending on age, overall health, and severity of symptoms. Some people don't require any treatment at all.

There are several methods to treat a UTI:

- Oral antibiotics – a type of antibiotic that is taken by mouth to treat an infection. Antibiotics have been around for more than 70 years and have greatly improved the health of millions of people around the world. However, sometimes they can cause side effects such as nausea, rash, or diarrhea. In certain cases, alternative treatment options may be preferable.
- Antibiotic creams – apply these near the infection site topically to relieve associated pain and discomfort caused by bacteria in the urine.
- Fluids – plenty of fluid consumption helps flush bacteria from the body.

- Over-the-counter medicines – e.g., Tylenol or ibuprofen to reduce fever and/or pain.
- Home remedies – such as drinking cranberry juice and increasing water intake and probiotics might help prevent UTIs. Although more study is needed, some research has suggested that cranberry juice might reduce the ability of bacteria to stick to urothelial cells in the urinary tract. The lack of scientific evidence means we don't know if these treatments can help get rid of a UTI or not.

What about alternative treatments for UTIs?

Some people use alternative treatments for UTIs, such as herbal remedies (e.g., goldenseal root), acetic acid, bismuth salts, or nitrofurantoin. More research is needed to determine if these are effective or not.

Some of these include:

Goldenseal root

Studies show conflicting results regarding the ability of goldenseal to treat UTIs. While some research shows it's no more effective than a placebo, other studies have found that it might be useful for the treatment of acute cystitis in women

Acetic acid

This acidic liquid is commonly used to kill bacteria, including those responsible for UTI infections. Studies suggest that acetic acid may be an effective method during pregnancy or in people with recurrent urinary tract infections

Bismuth subsalicylate

This salt-based compound contains two active ingredients: aspirin and bismuth (an element found naturally in rocks). It may affect the ability of bacteria to reproduce and spread in the body. However, more studies are needed to assess this treatment

Nitrofurantoin

This is an antibiotic that has been used for more than 50 years. However, one of its side effects is nausea, and, less frequently, it can lead to liver damage. Several UTIs caused by nitrofurantoin-resistant bacteria have also been reported

However, it's important to point out that there is currently no scientific evidence supporting the use of these alternative treatments.

Is there a way to prevent UTIs?

Women are more at risk for UTIs, in part because their urethra is shorter than that of a man's, making it easier for bacteria to reach the bladder. The following steps may help prevent UTIs:

- Drink plenty of fluids – If you're urinating every few hours it will help flush bacteria out of your urinary tract
- Urinate after sex – This can reduce the number of bacteria entering the urethra during intercourse
- Empty your bladder regularly – Don't hold urine for more than 4–5 hours as this increases the risk for urinary infections. Try to urinate every 2–3 hours during the day and 3-4 times per night. Moreover, pay attention to your urine color. If you feel like your urine is dark yellow, it means that the concentration of bacteria in your bladder might be high.
- Some women may benefit from taking an antibiotic before surgical procedures (i.e., before having teeth pulled) or after sexual intercourse as a preventative measure against UTI. However, this should only be done on a short-term basis and not for longer periods due to the risk of developing resistance to antibiotics over time.
- Keep genitals clean – Wash yourself daily with mild soap and water

The UTI Diet

Now that you have learned about UTIs, and their causes and prevention, you should start thinking about a UTI diet. Having a UTI can be annoying at best and painful at worst, but there are ways to cope with this infection so that your quality of life doesn't have to take a hit. The right UTI diet can help keep the pain at bay while speeding up recovery time.

In case you don't know much about what constitutes a UTI diet, food is not directly responsible for causing urinary tract infections.

However, poor eating habits can increase your susceptibility to getting an infection by making it easier for bacteria to thrive in your body. Also, certain foods might trigger an attack or make symptoms more intense since they cause changes in urine pH or irritate already inflamed tissues.

The most common UTI-triggering foods are (and thus should be avoided):

Caffeine

If you're sensitive to caffeine, it can cause your bladder muscle to contract more than needed. This will result in the irritating pain that's characteristic of having a UTI. Some examples of caffeine include coffee, black tea, green tea, and sodas

Sugar

Eating too much sugar can increase the risk for urinary tract infections because bacteria feed on this type of food. That said, only some types of bacteria cause UTIs so don't completely cut out desserts from your diet. But try to limit their consumption as much as you possibly can. Some examples of sugary foods include fruit juices, candies, and most processed foods

Alcohol

Alcoholic beverages also irritate already inflamed tissues and change urine pH, which may trigger an attack.

Foods high in acidity (e.g., tomatoes, citrus fruits, pineapple)

These types of food can also irritate the bladder and urethra, so it's best to avoid these types of foods.

Spicy foods

Many people experience an increase in bladder pain after eating spicy foods.

These are some good foods to eat:

Omega-3s

Studies have found out that people who get at least 600 milligrams of omega-3s per day lower their risk for urinary tract infections. Some types of fish rich in omega-3 fatty acids are sardines, herring, Pacific oysters, Atlantic mackerel, and Pacific halibut

Cranberry juice/extract

Diabetics often take cranberry juice supplements to counter the high levels of sugar in their blood. But drinking cranberries is also one way to lower your risk for UTIs. Cranberry juice and cranberry extracts can help keep bacteria that stick to your urinary tract walls away. Plus, they also inhibit bacterial growth.

Foods rich in vitamin C

Your body needs this nutrient for many different functions, including strengthening the walls of the bladder. So if you are prone to having recurrent UTI attacks, try to get more foods high in vitamin C into your diet. Some examples include oranges, watermelon, strawberries, kiwi fruit, blueberries, and red peppers

Foods with prebiotics

Prebiotics are fibers that promote the growth of good bacteria called "probiotics" in your gut. These probiotics help fight off potentially harmful microorganisms responsible for causing urinary tract infections. Some examples of prebiotics include:

- Asparagus
- artichoke
- chicory root
- garlic
- leek onion

Foods with probiotics

These are bacteria that are beneficial for your health, by helping keep the digestive system in balance. Lacto-fermented foods are one good source of probiotics. Some examples include yogurt, sauerkraut, and kimchi.

Asparagus

This is a great food to eat if you have recurrent UTIs because it can help clean your urinary tract by flushing out toxins. Just steam or grill it so you don't lose any of its nutrients. Alternatively, you can also drink asparagus juice by blending 1/2 cup of fresh chopped asparagus stems with 2 cups of water.

Water

This is extremely important for keeping your urinary tract healthy because it dilutes your urine and flushes out bacteria. Plus, it also keeps your urine at a more neutral pH level.

However, if you're prone to having UTIs often, then don't drink plain water because this can worsen the pain and inflammation in your bladder. Instead, try drinking decaffeinated tea or unsweetened cranberry juice. You can also add lemon to your pitcher of water or drink lukewarm water with a slice of lemon.

Whole grains

Research has found out that women who eat more whole grains, such as brown rice and oats, lower their risk for UTIs. Whole grains deliver prebiotics, which provide nourishment to the good bacteria already present in your gut that fight off harmful microorganisms.

Mushrooms

These are an excellent source of vitamin D, which your body needs to strengthen the walls of your bladder and urethra. Vitamin D also helps produce antimicrobial peptides that destroy harmful microorganisms. Just be sure to eat only the white button mushrooms because some other types can cause a sharp increase in urine acidity.

Watermelon

This is another good source of vitamin D, which can also help stop bacteria in their tracks. Just be sure to eat it raw because cooking or adding sugar to watermelon can reduce its beneficial effect.

Your 4-Step Plan for Managing UTIs

Now that you know the most important information about UTIs (causes, symptoms, and how they affect you), let's discuss the step-by-step plan for managing these infections. Here are the 4 key steps you'll need to follow:

Step 1: Keep your bladder healthy

If you want to prevent new UTIs, make sure you take care of your bladder first by following these tips:

Take some time to self-heal

Start practicing meditation and deep breathing exercises to relax. Think happy thoughts and try not to dwell on the pain that's constantly bothering you. Just keep reminding yourself that it's all going to be fine soon enough.

Vitamin C therapy

Take some vitamin C supplements or opt for more foods rich in this nutrient if you have a history of recurrent UTIs. Vitamin C is useful for strengthening the walls of your urinary tract, so an increased intake can help reinforce them against bacteria trying to invade it.

Step 2: Prevent bacteria from building up in your urinary tract

Do whatever you can to prevent bacteria from entering your urinary tract. Here are some tips on how to do that:

Maintain a healthy weight

Obesity is linked to an increased risk of developing UTIs, so losing extra pounds gives you one less thing to worry about. Be sure to eat more fruits and vegetables and drink 8 glasses of water every day. Also make it a priority to be physically active because exercise helps speed up your metabolism, allowing the toxins in your body (including any existing bacteria) to move out faster. It also enables you to shed excess pounds better and more effectively.

Avoid wearing tight-fitted pants/jeans

Tight clothing such as skinny jeans or tight pants (especially when they're made of denim material) can cause skin irritation, which makes it easier for bacteria to invade your urinary tract. If you feel more comfortable wearing them during the colder months, make sure to change into loose-fitting clothes or skirts when you get inside the house or return home after taking care of errands.

Take antibiotics only when necessary

Antibiotics kill off both good and bad bacteria in your body. When this happens, it gives room for harmful microorganisms that are known to cause UTIs to have an upper hand because there are fewer of them to keep them away. Use antibiotics only when you need them. This applies especially if you take high doses of these medications regularly so be mindful of your dosage.

Step 3: Manage urinary tract infections

If you already have a UTI, here are the steps on how to manage it properly:

Fluid intake

Drinking more water is one of the best things you can do for your bladder because bacteria thrive in an environment where there's less urine present. As mentioned earlier, aim to take 8 glasses of water every day. Increase this amount if you're taking diuretic medications or if it's hot and humid outside. Also avoid drinks that act as diuretics such as coffee, tea, alcohol, and sodas. These beverages dehydrate your body so instead opt for healthier choices like coconut juice or green tea to keep yourself hydrated throughout the day.

Probiotics

Taking probiotic supplements not only helps introduce good bacteria into your system but also aids in managing UTIs by reducing inflammation and pain. Try taking 10 billion colony-forming units (CFU) every day through capsules or powders.

Step 4: Eat a UTI-friendly Diet

As mentioned in the previous chapter, make sure you follow the guidelines on what foods to eat and what foods to avoid for UTIs. Here is an example meal plan idea that is healthy:

- Breakfast: 1 glass of water and a bowl of oatmeal with blueberries and strawberries.
- Lunch: A piece of baked salmon, quinoa salad, and broccoli soup.
- Dinner: Brown rice pasta with basil pesto sauce and butternut squash soup.
- Snack Time: Apple slices dipped in almond butter or yogurt mixed with berries as your healthy snack for the day.

By doing this, you will be able to eat healthily and lessen your chances of getting UTIs in the future.

Sample Recipes

Garlic Broccoli Salad

Ingredients:

- 1 head broccoli, cut into florets
- 1 tsp. olive oil
- 1-1/2 tbsp. rice wine vinegar
- 1 tbsp. sesame oil
- 2 cloves garlic, minced
- 1 pinch cayenne pepper
- 3 tbsp. golden raisins

Instructions:

1. Fill water into a steamer. Bring to a boil.
2. Add broccoli. Cover. Steam until tender for about 3 minutes.
3. Rinse broccoli and set aside.
4. Heat olive oil in a skillet over medium heat.
5. Put in pine nuts. Stir fry for 1-2 minutes.
6. Remove from heat.
7. Whisk together rice vinegar, sesame oil, pepper, and garlic.
8. Transfer the broccoli, nuts, and raisins to the rice vinegar dressing.
9. Serve and enjoy.

Grenade Salad

Ingredients:

- 4 cups arugula
- 1 large avocado
- 1/2 cup sliced fennel
- 1/2 cup sliced Anjou pears
- /4 cup pomegranate seeds

Instructions:

1. Mix all the ingredients except for the pomegranate seeds.
2. After mixing well, add the seeds. Mix again.
3. Serve with any type of desired dressing.

Spinach and Watercress Salad

Ingredients:

- 1 cup watercress, washed with stems removed
- 3 cups baby spinach, washed with stems removed
- 1 medium sliced avocado
- 1/4 cup avocado oil
- 1/8 cup lemon juice
- a pinch of salt

Instructions:

1. Pat dry the spinach and watercress. Remove the stem and separate the leaves.
2. On a large serving plate, combine the leaves of the watercress and the spinach.
3. Cut the avocado in half, then remove the pit. Peel the skin off from each side.
4. Slice the avocados into thin strips. Set aside.
5. Prepare the dressing by combining avocado oil and lemon juice.
6. Arrange the avocado strips on top of the watercress and spinach.
7. Season with salt and pepper.
8. Drizzle with the dressing before serving.

Kale Salad with Strawberry and Almonds

Ingredients:

- 1 bunch of kale
- 1/2 cup sliced strawberries
- 1/4 cup sliced almonds
- 1 lemon pulp juice
- 1/8 tsp. salt
- 1/8 tsp. black pepper
- 1 tbsp. agave
- 2 tbsp. of olive oil

Instructions:

1. Rip kale into small pieces and massage with hands until tender.
2. Put it in a bowl. Add almonds and strawberries.
3. To create a dressing, mix lemon juice with olive oil, salt, pepper, and agave, and then pour it over the salad.
4. Serve immediately.

Roasted Veggies

Ingredients:

- 1/2 lb. turnips
- 1/2 lb. carrots
- 1/2 lb. parsnips
- 2 shallots, peeled
- 1/4 tsp. ground black pepper
- 1 tbsp. extra-virgin olive oil
- 6 cloves garlic
- 3/4 tsp. kosher salt
- 2 tbsp. fresh rosemary needles

Instructions:

1. First, cut vegetables into bite-sized pieces.
2. Set the oven to 400°F.
3. Mix all the ingredients in a baking dish.
4. Roast the vegetables for 25 minutes until brown and tender.
5. Toss and roast again for 20–25 minutes.
6. Serve and enjoy while hot.

Coleslaw

Ingredients:

- 1/2 cup virgin olive oil
- 1/2 head of red cabbage, chopped into small pieces
- 1 head of green cabbage, chopped into small pieces
- 1 tsp. unrefined sea salt, finely ground
- 2 green onions, chopped
- 4 drops organic stevia
- 8 organic carrots, shredded
- optional: a bunch of cilantro, chopped
- optional: 1 green apple, chopped finely

Instructions:

1. Mix all the chopped vegetables.
2. Blend in salt, virgin olive oil, and stevia together using a whisk or a blender.
3. Pour the blended slaw into the mixed vegetables.
4. Add apples upon serving.

Seafood Stew

Ingredients:

- 2 tsp. extra-virgin olive oil
- 1 cut bulb fennel
- 2 stalks celery, chopped
- 2 cups white wine
- 1 tbsp. chopped thyme
- 1 cup chopped shallots
- 6 ounces shrimp
- 6 ounces of sea scallops
- 1/4 tsp. salt
- 1 cup chopped parsley
- 6 oz. Arctic char
- 2-1/2 cups of water

Instructions:

1. Heat a frying pan on the lowest setting. Add a small amount of oil.
2. Cook the celery, shallots, and fennel for approximately 6 minutes.
3. Pour the wine, water, and thyme into the frying pan.
4. Wait for 10 minutes and allow it to cook.
5. Once much of the water has evaporated, add in the remaining ingredients, and wait for 2 minutes before removing it from the stove.
6. Serve and enjoy immediately.

Baked Tuna and Asparagus

Ingredients:

- 2 5-oz. tuna fillets
- 14 oz. young potatoes
- 8 asparagus spears, trimmed and halved
- 2 handfuls of cherry tomatoes
- 1 handful fresh basil leaves
- 2 tbsp. extra-virgin olive oil
- 1 tbsp. balsamic vinegar

Instructions:

1. Heat oven to 428°F.
2. Arrange potatoes in a baking dish. Drizzle with a tablespoon of extra-virgin olive oil.
3. Roast potatoes for 20 minutes, or until golden brown.
4. Place the asparagus into the baking dish together with the potatoes. Roast in the oven for another 15 minutes.
5. Arrange the cherry tomatoes and tuna among the vegetables. Drizzle with balsamic vinegar and the remaining olive oil.
6. Roast for 10 to 15 minutes, or until tuna is cooked.
7. Throw in a handful of basil leaves before transferring everything to a serving dish. Serve while hot.

Baked Salmon

Ingredients:

- 2 salmon fillets
- 6 cups of fresh spinach
- 2 tsp. coconut oil
- 1/4 tsp. garlic powder
- 1/4 tsp. turmeric
- 3 large cloves of garlic
- lemon juice
- salt
- pepper

Instructions:

1. Preheat the oven to 400°F.
2. Line a baking dish with parchment paper.
3. Marinate salmon fillets in lemon juice, coconut oil, garlic powder, turmeric, salt, and pepper.
4. Let it sit for a few minutes. This may also be done the night before to help the juices and flavor get into the salmon.
5. Once the oven is ready, bake salmon for 15 minutes.
6. Cook some of the garlic in a pan with coconut oil.
7. Add spinach and cook until ready. Season with salt and pepper to taste.
8. Take salmon out of the oven and put spinach beside it.
9. Serve and enjoy.

Garbanzo-Kale and Butternut Squash Burger

Ingredients:

- 1/2 cup brown rice
- 1/2 cup quinoa

Beetroot burger:

- 2 cups kale, chopped
- 1 tsp. paprika
- 1 cup butternut squash, chopped
- 1/2 cup sauerkraut, bottled
- 3/4 cup garbanzo beans
- 2 tbsp. coconut oil
- 1 tsp. sea salt

Instructions:

1. In a pan, boil quinoa and water. Cook for 20 minutes. Set aside
2. Combine kale and butternut squash in a small bowl.
3. Add the paprika, garbanzo beans, sea salt, and coconut oil.
4. Sauté the mixture until vegetables soften.
5. Prepare the burger by making balls. Flatten the burger and fry until done.
6. Use quinoa and rice as buns for the burger.
7. Serve on a plate and enjoy!

Lentil Soup

Ingredients:

- 1 tbsp. avocado oil
- 1 cup onion, diced
- 1/2 cup carrot, diced
- 1/2 cup celery, diced
- 4 cups vegetable or chicken broth
- 1 cup dried red lentils, well rinsed
- 1/4 tsp dried thyme
- 1/2 cup fresh flat-leaf parsley, chopped
- salt and pepper, to taste

Instructions:

1. Sauté carrot, celery and onion in a large saucepan over medium heat. Do so until they are soft.
2. Pour in the broth with lentils and thyme and wait to boil.
3. Lower the heat. Cover and leave to simmer until lentils are soft, about 20 minutes.
4. Transfer the soup to a blender.
5. Set the blender on high. Purée the soup until it's creamy.
6. If it's too thick, pour in a cup of water.
7. Add salt and pepper to taste.

8. Return to the saucepan to reheat if necessary.
9. Ladle into bowls and garnish with parsley.
10. Serve and enjoy while hot.

Vegetable Broth

Ingredients:

- 1 tbsp. oil
- 2 leeks, sliced
- 2 carrots, sliced
- 2 ribs celery
- 1/4 tsp. salt
- 8 cups water

To make the soup:

- 1 tbsp. oil
- 2 cups potatoes, diced
- 1 cup mushrooms, diced
- 1-1/2 cups cauliflower, diced
- 1 cup onion, diced
- 1 cup celery, diced
- 1 cup carrot, diced
- 1-1/2 cups red beans, cooked
- 2 sprigs rosemary
- 4 sprigs thyme
- 2 cups spinach

Instructions:

1. To a pot on medium heat, add oil and leeks.
2. Cook for about three minutes or until they start to soften up.

3. Add carrots and top a few celery stalks with leaves.
4. Cover with water.
5. Add salt. Bring to a simmer and cook until carrots are very tender but not mushy.
6. Turn off the heat and let it cool down a little.
7. When the broth has cooled down, strain out the veggies.
8. Remove carrots and set them aside.
9. Squeeze most of the liquid out of the leeks and celery.

To cook the soup:

1. Add carrots to some of the broth and blend.
2. With a pot on medium heat, add oil, onions, raw carrots, and celery. Cook until onions are translucent, approximately 3 to 5 minutes.
3. Add broth, potatoes, and herbs.
4. Bring to a simmer and cook for 10 minutes.
5. Add cauliflower and red beans.
6. Simmer for another 5 minutes.
7. Add the package of frozen green beans and cook until the potatoes and cauliflower are tender, approximately for another 5 minutes.
8. At the end of cooking, add spinach.
9. Serve warm.

Zucchini and Celery Greens Soup

Ingredients:

- 1/2 cup cooked green lentils
- 1 onion, finely diced
- 1 parsnip, peeled and finely diced
- 2 garlic cloves, crushed
- 1 green bell pepper, cut into small cubes
- 1 zucchini, sliced
- 4 asparagus spears
- 1 fennel bulb, diced finely
- 2 celery stalks, diced finely
- 1 small bunch of celery greens or other greens available: beet greens, kale, or spinach
- 2 cups low sodium vegetable broth
- 1 lime, juice only
- 1 tsp. chia seeds to garnish
- freshly ground black pepper

Instructions:

1. Stir-fry onion and garlic, about 2 minutes.
2. Throw in the parsnip, bell pepper, fennel, celery stalks, and zucchini, along with the vegetable broth.
3. Wait until it boils. Then, lower the heat and let it simmer for 7 minutes.

4. Put in the asparagus, lime juice, lentils, and celery greens. Turn off the heat.
5. Serve warm, garnished with chia seeds.

Energy Oats

Ingredients:

- 1 cup rolled oats
- 1 tbsp. walnuts
- 1 tbsp. flaxseed
- 1 tbsp. almonds, sliced
- 1 cup blueberries or fruit of choice
- 1 cup almond or soy milk

Instructions:

1. Combine oats, nuts, seeds, and milk.
2. Soak for 5 minutes.
3. Microwave on medium-low for 1-2 minutes or until the oats are tender.
4. Add in fruit.
5. Serve while warm.

Spinach Quiche

Ingredients:

- 1 lb. breakfast sausage
- 1/2 onion, diced
- 2 cups mushrooms, sliced
- 6 cups spinach, roughly chopped
- 12 eggs
- 1/4 to 1/2 cup full-fat coconut milk
- 1 tsp. garlic powder
- 1 tsp. Italian seasoning
- 1 tsp. salt
- 1 tsp. pepper

Instructions:

1. Preheat the oven to 400°F.
2. Heat a cast-iron pan or another oven-safe pan over medium heat.
3. Cook sausage and onion. Stir occasionally until sausage turns brown, about 7-8 minutes.
4. Add in mushrooms. Allow them to cook with the sausage until soft, for about 2 minutes. Remove from heat.
5. Crack eggs into a large bowl.
6. Add coconut milk. For a lighter and fluffier texture, use ½ cup. Use less for less coconut taste.
7. Whisk together well to get a light egg mixture.

8. Add spinach and seasonings to the bowl with the eggs.
9. Add the sausage mixture to the bowl with the rest of the ingredients.
10. Mix until everything is well blended.
11. Line the pan with some fat from the sausage or grease well with oil, butter, or ghee to prevent the quiche from sticking.
12. Pour the mixture into the cast iron pan or oven-safe dish.
13. Bake for 40-45 minutes or until a knife poked at the center comes out clean.
14. Serve and enjoy while warm.

Salmon and Fennel Salad

Ingredients:

- 4 pcs. skinless salmon filets
- 2 tsp. parsley, chopped finely
- 1 tsp. thyme, chopped finely
- 2 tbsp. olive oil
- 4 cups fennel, sliced
- 1 clove garlic clove, grated
- 2 tbsp. orange juice
- 1 tsp. lemon juice
- 2/3 cup greek yogurt
- 2 tbsp. dill, chopped

Instructions:

1. Preheat the oven to 200°F.
2. Take a small bowl, and add the thyme and parsley. Stir them well.
3. Put the salmon over a flat surface and brush some oil. Sprinkle the mixed herb mixture evenly.
4. Place 2 filets at a time in the air fryer basket. Cook them for 10 minutes at 350°F.
5. Once done, transfer them to the preheated oven to keep warm. Repeat the process with the remaining salmon filets.

6. In a medium-sized bowl, add the sliced fennel along with grated garlic, yogurt, dill, lemon juice, orange juice, and remaining salt. Toss them well.
7. Serve the filets hot over the fennel salad.

Marinated Tuna Steak

Ingredients:

- 4 slices tuna steak
- 1/3 cup soy sauce
- 1 tbsp. cider vinegar
- 3 tbsp. olive oil
- 2 tbsp. chopped parsley
- 1 tbsp. chopped rosemary
- 1/2 tsp. chopped oregano
- 1/8 tsp. garlic powder

Instructions:

1. Put together olive oil, soy sauce, parsley, cider vinegar, rosemary, and oregano in a bowl. Mix well to create a marinade mixture.
2. Using a gallon plastic bag, put tuna steaks and marinade mixture. Allow the mixture to coat the tuna by turning the bag over.
3. Leave inside the refrigerator for 30 minutes.
4. Put a small amount of oil on the grill grate. Cook tuna for about 5 minutes per side.
5. Put some of the remaining marinade mixtures on the tuna every few minutes.

Creamy Low-FODMAP Fish Casserole

Ingredients:

- 1-1/2 lb. white fish, serving-sized pieces
- 2 tbsp. olive oil
- 2 tbsp. small capers
- 1 lb. broccoli
- 1 oz. grass-fed butter
- 6 scallions
- 1 tbsp. Dijon mustard
- 1 tbsp. dried barley
- 1 tsp. salt
- 1/4 tsp. ground black pepper*

Instructions:

1. Set the oven temperature to 400°F.
2. Cut the broccoli into small florets with the stems included. Fry the broccoli for 3-5 minutes until soft and golden, then add salt and pepper.
3. Add the finely chopped scallions and the capers, then fry for another 2-3 minutes.
4. Grease the baking dish with butter and add in the fried vegetables.
5. Add the white fish to the vegetable mix.
6. In an oven-ready plate, mix the parsley, mustard, and whipping cream. Add the fish and vegetable mix and top with some butter.

7. Bake for 20-30 minutes or until fully cooked then serve.
8. In this particular recipe, broccoli is considered a high-FODMAP vegetable.

*black pepper may be substituted with white pepper

Conclusion

Having a UTI, especially when it's recurring, can be a very frustrating experience. Aside from the pain and discomfort, being repeatedly diagnosed with having one may require you to visit the doctor frequently and retake antibiotics, which can be very costly.

Following a diet that may aid in lessening this burden and even benefit your overall health further, can prove to be extremely helpful.

The UTI Diet is a good program to follow to help you avoid a recurring UTI diagnosis. Doing this along with sticking to a healthier, more active lifestyle can greatly benefit you, not only to help ease the symptoms of UTIs but may also improve your life. Just make sure that you consult with your doctor first before starting and sticking to these types of programs.

We hope that you have enjoyed this short quick-start guide on how to manage UTIs through diet. We wish you all the best in your endeavors. If you have found this content valuable, please leave a review.

References and Helpful Links

CDC. (2022, January 14). Suffering from a urinary tract infection? Centers for Disease Control and Prevention. https://www.cdc.gov/antibiotic-use/uti.html.

Urinary tract infection (Uti)—Symptoms and causes. (n.d.). Mayo Clinic. Retrieved November 27, 2022, from https://www.mayoclinic.org/diseases-conditions/urinary-tract-infection/symptoms-causes/syc-20353447.

What to eat (and avoid) during a UTI. (2021, February 2). DispatchHealth. https://www.dispatchhealth.com/blog/what-to-eat-and-avoid-during-uti/.

What to eat (and what to avoid) during a UTI. (n.d.). Retrieved November 27, 2022, from https://www.eehealth.org/blog/2019/05/what-to-eat-during-a-uti/.

www.ingramcontent.com/pod-product-compliance
Lightning Source LLC
LaVergne TN
LVHW051924060526
838201LV00062B/4676